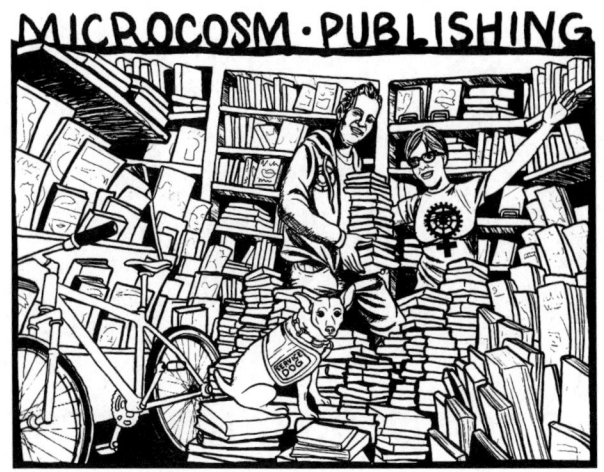

Microcosm Publishing is Portland's most diversified publishing house and distributor with a focus on the colorful, authentic, and empowering. Our books and zines have put your power in your hands since 1996, equipping readers to make positive changes in their lives and in the world around them. Microcosm emphasizes skill-building, showing hidden histories, and fostering creativity through challenging conventional publishing wisdom with books and bookettes about DIY skills, food, bicycling, gender, self-care, and social justice. What was once a distro and record label started by Joe Biel in a drafty bedroom was determined to be *Publishers Weekly*'s fastest-growing publisher of 2022 and has become among the oldest independent publishing houses in Portland, OR, and Cleveland, OH. We are a politically moderate, centrist publisher in a world that has inched to the right for the past 80 years.

For Becca, who first told me "It's way more than Kegels," and whose careful editorial eye helped bring this booklet to life.

INTRODUCTION

We all have a pelvic floor. It is the layers of muscles that sit within the pelvic girdle of your skeleton. We often only think about it when there's a problem or perhaps occasionally during excretion or sex. However, the Pelvic Floor Musculature (PFM) plays important structural and functional roles in our bodies.

When the pelvic floor muscles are restricted, other muscles in your legs and back are painfully forced to attempt to compensate for its lack of mobility. Over time if your pelvic floor muscles are constantly tensed, you'll find that you cannot hold your bladder and will eventually be in chronic pain, which can result in numerous diagnoses.

While everyone has a pelvic floor, I am a woman with female anatomy, so my personal anecdotes stem from that. While women are more likely to experience chronic conditions related to the pelvic floor, people of all sexes and genders suffer from these conditions and can benefit from education about the Pelvic Floor Musculature (PFM) and how posture and neuroanatomy contribute to its functioning.

It is never too early nor too late to learn about your pelvic floor and neuromuscular functioning. You can start today to educate yourself and adopt habits that will support your PFM each day and for years to come.

If you are in pain, I wish you hope and strength as you find good practitioners. Know that I'm rooting for you on your journey and glad this educational booklet might be of use on that journey. If you're not in pain you can develop supportive habits to keep it that way in your daily life!

Clinical evidence shows that one of the most effective treatments for long-term success in managing chronic pelvic pain is education about the body (Philip, 2016). When we learn about our bodies and *how* particular exercises and approaches support them, we're more likely to do the exercises and to feel like we have control over our condition and can work toward managing it. Health practitioners and movement and bodywork professionals are starting to bring information on the pelvic floor, fascia, neurophysiology, and chronic pain to the mainstream, and scientists are conducting more clinical studies on these issues and the connections between them. Understanding our bodies and integrating that knowledge with our minds and the world around us not only supports our physical health, but empowers us to make changes that can have lasting positive impacts on many facets of our lives.

If you are suffering from chronic pain or other issues, please see a medical practitioner to assess your personal situation. However, be warned that good care does not always equal good treatment. The modern medical system is not designed to approach chronic pain in a holistic way; referrals from general practitioner to specialist to physical therapist back to general practitioner are all too common, and doctors are often not given the time to educate their patients in a way they might like. That is why I present this material as a supplement in order to better understand how that knowledge is empowerment.

Keep moving, but go slow,

-awj

BASIC PELVIC FLOOR ANATOMY

*T*he PFM is roughly diamond shaped, spanning from the pubic bone in front, back to the tailbone, and bordered by the sitting bones. The pelvic floor muscles support the pelvic organs, resist abdominal pressure, and work as sphincters, opening and closing the urethra, rectum, and vagina.

Different descriptions categorize the PFM muscles in different ways; some say it's three layers of muscle, some refer to it as 2 muscle groups, and some call it a diaphragm, as it spans a large area. The most important takeaway from these differences is to know that it is a complex group of muscles and their supportive connective tissues. It is not like your bicep which contracts and relaxes along one plane, moving one bone. It includes larger muscles that span the "diamond" for support as well as smaller sphincter muscles that control the openings in the pelvic floor. Like other skeletal muscle, the muscles that make up the PFM are supported by a variety of ligaments and connective tissue fascia interwoven between them.

What the heck is fascia? Fascia is a thin membrane of connective tissue that wraps around each bundle of muscles. It functions throughout every single part of the body—from lining large cavities to wrapping tiny capillaries—providing support and maintaining divisions between organs, blood vessels, and other tissues. If you've ever broken down a chicken, you've experienced fascia.

For the veg crowd, you can think of it like the thin membrane that separates each segment of an orange (Open Hand Health, 2021). It's strong and supportive, but you can easily tear it apart. Like ligaments and other connective tissue, fascia is made up of fibers. Fascia is largely collagen, which provides more strength than stretch. Collagen in your body needs to be used and moved in order to stay lubricated and pliable. Damage or lack of use can lead to a stiffening of the muscle it surrounds and stiffness in the overall area of the body.

In your PFM there are multiple layers of fascia, which wrap and support the layers of the PFM and connect it to surrounding areas, such as uterine ligaments. Tasha Mulligan, a physical therapist who specializes in pelvic health, suggests thinking of the PFM as a basket (Mulligan, 2013). The various interwoven parts provide support for the structure and functioning of the PFM. We'll come back to this basket imagery when we talk about strengthening.

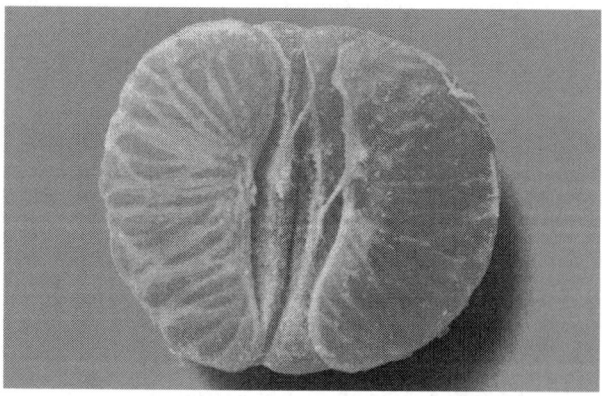

Photo of orange segments by Charles Deluvio on Unsplash

MUSCLES OF THE PFM

The levator ani is a large muscle, made up of the pubococcygeus and the iliococcygeus. Some consider the levator ani the most important muscle of the pelvic floor because it supports the organs within the pelvis. It also provides the lift that resists pressure produced by contraction of the abdominal muscles, such as that created during exercise, birth, defecating, or coughing. A healthy levator ani will automatically contract in response to pressure from these activities. It's also the muscle most likely to sustain damage, particularly during childbirth (Bo et al., 2015). Along with its supportive role, the levator ani creates skeletal muscle sphincters at the urethra and anus.

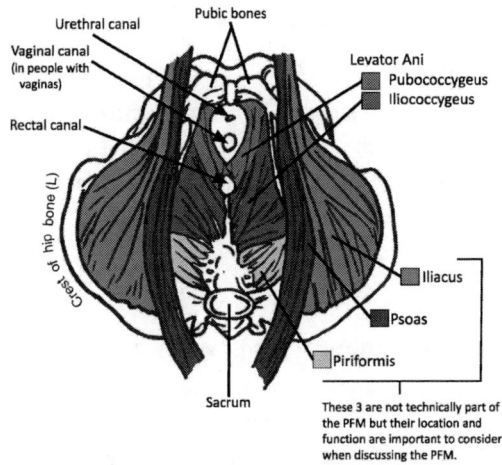

Figure 1.1—Muscles of the Pelvic Floor from above, looking down on the diamond shape.

The bulbospongiosus and ischiocavernosus muscles are located toward the front of the PFM. They compress to support urination as well as supporting erectile tissue in both males and females.

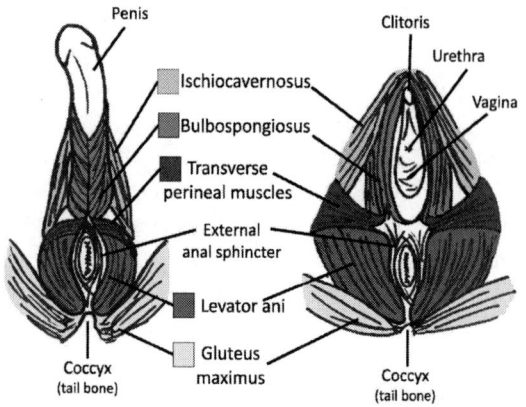

Figure 1.2—Muscles of the pelvic floor and perineum from below, showing a comparison between male and female anatomy

Muscles of the perineum (that space between the genitals and anus) provide support for the PFM and the function of the sphincters. The perineal muscles include both superficial and deep layers, with some differences in male and female anatomy. Additional muscles, called the compressor urethra and sphincter urethrovaginalis, function to close the vagina. In males, the deep transverse perineal muscle plays a role in ejaculation.

MUSCLES THAT SUPPORT THE PFM

Because your legs and trunk also stem from the pelvic girdle, these muscles are important to pelvic floor health. Maintaining strength in your abdominal muscles, hip muscles, low back muscles, and inner thighs can help support your PFM.

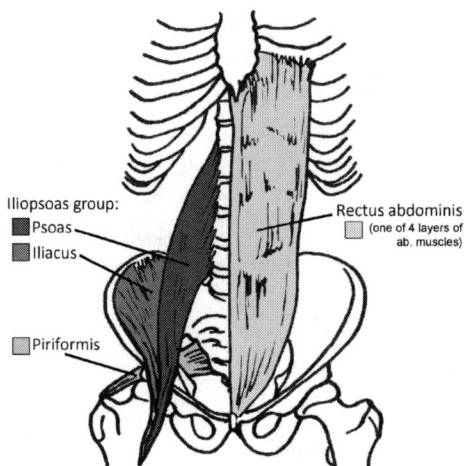

Figure 1.3—View from the front: Muscles that stem from and support the pelvic girdle play a role in the functioning of the PFM

The following describes how other muscle groups work with and support the PFM:

Abdominals (abs)—These four layers of muscles have multiple roles including postural support, movement, and protection of abdominal organs. They have attachment points on the pelvic girdle. Contraction of the abs puts pressure on the PFM.

Glutes—Notoriously the largest muscle group in your body, these are responsible for keeping you upright and extending your legs. Also play a major role in stabilizing the hips and pelvis.

Piriformis—Located under your glutes, this band connects your sacrum to the top of your femur. Because it supports the sacrum, any damage or tension in it creates tension in the pelvic floor (Philip, 2016).

Iliopsoas—This group includes the *iliacus,* a flat triangular muscle originating along the crest of the hip bone and extending down to the inside of the femur, and the *psoas,* a long muscle extending all the way from the thoracic and lumbar spine down to the inside of your femur. The group's main function is as a hip flexor, bringing your leg up. It also plays a role in maintaining posture and in side-bending. Tightness in the iliopsoas can also cause pain in the PFM.

Multifidus—This muscle/muscle group extends along your spine attaching to each vertebral segment. It coordinates with the other core muscles (pelvic floor and abs) to provide stability. Weakness in any of the core muscles can lead to low back or pelvic pain.

Obturator internus—Rotates the thigh from side to side. If damaged, pain can be felt in the groin and glutes (Philip, 2016).

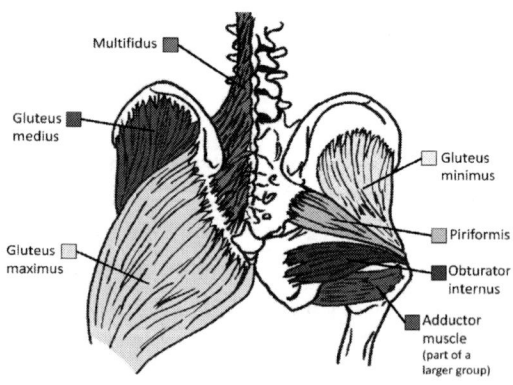

Figure 1.4—View from the back: Muscles that stem from and support the pelvic girdle play a role in the functioning of the PFM

In order to support and care for your pelvic floor it's important to keep in mind that this complex group of muscles and connective tissue is performing multiple roles and is connected to and affected by other muscle groups. As skeletal muscle, it can be strengthened, but there are supportive and unsupportive ways to approach this. Simple habits related to alignment and movement can help support and keep the Pelvic Floor Muscles and connective tissue balanced, responsive, and functioning without pain.

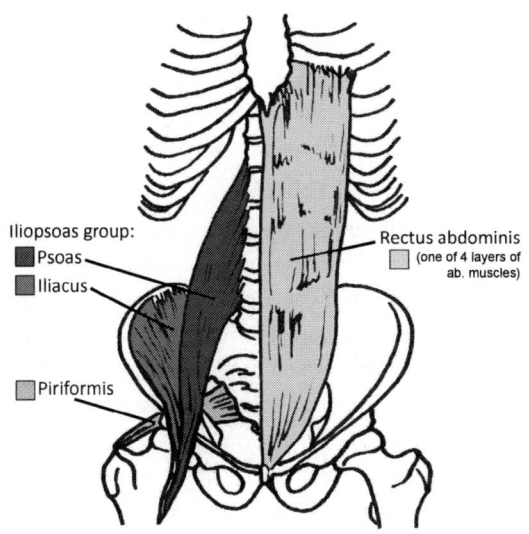

YOUR POSTURE AND YOUR PELVIC FLOOR

The pelvic floor is integrated into the pelvic girdle of your skeleton. The sacrum anchors the base of your spine, supporting the entire spinal column all the way up through your neck. Your spine is essential to understand because *every* sensation you feel as well as *every* command you give in response to sensation goes through your spine. Therefore, when things aren't functioning properly in your pelvic floor, it often means they're not functioning properly in your sensory system.

The spinal column is important for supporting you and providing spaces for nerves to pass in and out, but it's also the attachment site for many muscles and ligaments. If it's out of alignment, it will stretch and pull on these muscles and ligaments, which over time can cause some to become deconditioned (weak from disuse) while others become too tight. Both of these conditions can lead to pain because of how they impact nerves. Over time, your nerves can change in response to constant irregular stimulation, whether it's from being compressed, from chronic inflammation, or other inputs triggering them (Philip, 2016).

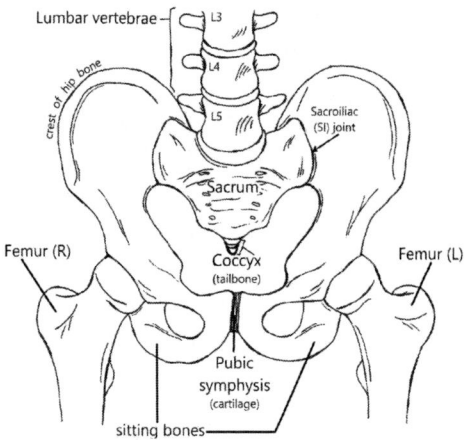

Figure 2.1—View from the front of how the sacrum is anchored in the pelvic girdle.

Back issues and pelvic pain often become chronic. The symptoms may seem like they came on all of a sudden, but it likely took a long time of bad positioning, holding tension, and habitual cycles to get to the point of pain. This means it will take time to address these habits and relieve the pain. While many of us are familiar with the idea that poor posture can lead to neck pain, shoulder pain, back pain, and other problems, we're often not thinking about how poor posture affects the pelvic floor. Posture is all about balance, and when this balance is off, it alters our alignment, shifting muscle tension and negatively affecting joints and muscles (Philip, 2016).

Visualizing supportive posture is the first step to understanding how posture supports your PFM. The goal for your posture should be to maintain a "neutral spine." This is when each of the natural curves of the spine balance each other out in order to be supportive and reduce load (see figure 2.2). In this position, muscles are engaged, but not tense, and provide support from the pelvic girdle all the way up to the skull.

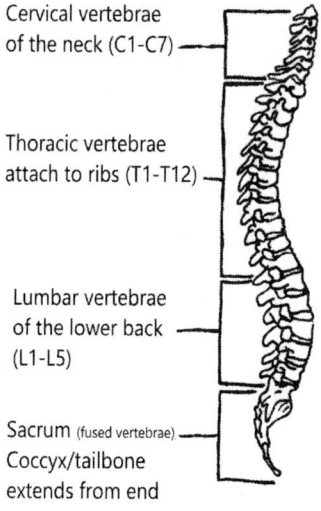

Figure 2.2—A side view of the spine, showing its natural curves.

When thinking about poor posture, we often think about slouching. Slouching puts strain on your spine all the way down. It also disengages muscles that support the spine. As these muscles become deconditioned, nerves get pinched, pulled, or otherwise damaged, leading to pain.

However, poor posture can also result from standing or moving in any exaggerated way, even from postures we've taken on as an attempt to stand up straight. Many of us try to bring elements of "proper" posture into our daily lives, emulating ballet posture with abs engaged and bottom tucked or gymnast posture with shoulders pushed back and an accentuated lumbar curve. Both of these examples put stress on the spine and affect the positioning and engagement of everything else attached to the spine, especially the pelvic floor.

As an example, Mulligan encourages taking a minute to notice what happens when you lock your knees (Mulligan, 2013). Many of us, thinking it's part of good posture, stand super erect with our knees locked. Try standing up with fully straight locked knees. Now relax your knees just a little and make a mental note of how your pelvis feels and how it is tilted in relation to the rest of your alignment. Now lock your knees again and notice what your pelvis does. Did you notice your pelvis tilt? You also may have noticed a ripple effect of tightening in your upper back or your shoulders moving forward just a touch to balance the tilt of your pelvis. These changes feel minor, but over time they can cause problems. When your hips move forward tilting the pelvis back, you disengage the PFM while also taking away its skeletal support. This puts increased pressure on the PFM as well as strain on nearby ligaments and bones. The consequences are especially bad for anyone with bladder prolapse or other PFM dysfunction (Mulligan, 2013).

Posture correction often focuses on lumbar support and maintaining a lumbar curve. However, overexaggerating the lumbar curve can cause the hip bones to tilt too far forward, causing the PFM to be constantly stretched tight. When muscles are held in a tight position for extended periods of time, blood flow may be restricted, which can cause pain (Bo et al., 2015). With the muscle fibers stretched tight it also becomes harder for the muscles to contract, contributing to weakness or atrophy. Forward-tilting of the hips also over-stretches the transversus abdominus muscle across the front of our pelvis, and disengages the multifidus muscles that run along the lower back and sacrum (Mulligan, 2013). Over time these shifts can lead to asymmetry in the tilt of the pelvis as well as the way the muscles hold tension. These factors can become painful as they affect functioning of the lower spine and abdominal muscles (Philip, 2016).

As an example of how posture can affect the body over time, think about alignment in a pregnant body. Many pregnant people develop posture-related back pain. Rapid weight gain causes a shift to their center of gravity, affecting alignment. On top of that, changes in hormones cause ligaments to become looser, which affects the engagement of the abdominals and the stabilization of the pelvis. This is an accelerated example of what can happen to *all of us* over time. As we age, many of us put on weight, and we all have changes in hormones that affect our tissues. Many of us, consciously or unconsciously, have also taken on protective postures which lead to a stiffening in the muscles and fascia (Philip, 2016). This can become chronic pain due to tightness or other issues in the PFM and related muscles. Studies show that in patients with chronic pelvic pain, persistent tightness is also often present in the lumbar muscles and hip flexors (Kisner, 2018).

Maintaining neutral posture will not only support your back and neck, but also support your PFM and help you keep moving comfortably throughout your life. One study even found that education in neutral spine alignment facilitated the healing process of *all* pelvic pain patients, regardless of what their physiological issue was (Philip, 2016). The researchers thought this was partly due to patients feeling empowered to self correct; it probably also helped that they were paying attention to their alignment and thereby getting biofeedback about how the muscles relate to each other. Remember, the first step to addressing your posture is paying attention to what your spine is doing. As you pay attention, you'll notice that maintaining neutral posture supports your spine and actually requires less energy and muscle tension than trying to push into and hold "proper" upright posture (Essential Somatics, 2019).

"ENGAGING MY CORE" WRECKED MY PELVIC FLOOR.

In the years following the birth of my large-headed baby, I received no suggestions or instruction in pelvic rehab from multiple professionals, including a gynecologist who told me directly there was nothing I could do about it unless I wanted a hysterectomy, "Haha." I figured I just had to learn to live with minor bladder prolapse. I didn't even think it was an issue when I took on a baking job in a cafe. However, this particular job had me working in the basement—carrying equipment and heavy trays up and down stairs. I thought "engaging my abs" and tucking under to engage my glutes would help, but within two months my prolapse was significantly worse, and I was in terrible pain with muscle spasms throughout my PFM and abs. I felt like a bomb had gone off in my pelvis. One gynecologist did an exam and ultrasound and "couldn't see anything" that was causing the pain. Another gynecologist fortunately knew about spasms and prescribed me physical therapy. My PT addressed my muscle imbalances and showed me how to properly contract my PFM. Further reading taught me to pay attention to my posture and work to engage my PFM properly in my daily activities.

As I learned about the neutral spine, I found that the "protective posture" I was taking on was actually contributing to the problem. As I squeezed my glutes and abs, it tilted my pelvis back putting pressure on my PFM while also taking away the skeletal support that is typically below it. That movement, combined with carrying 30 pounds of dough up the stairs multiple times a day, significantly weakened and likely damaged my PFM, causing it to revolt in the pain that spread through my abdomen. Most days I still have some pain—I'm working to address chronic tension and likely have residual nervous system effects. However, learning about my body has empowered me to understand and manage my condition. Along with less pain, I've seen some reversal in my prolapse. I've even noticed that slowing down to pay attention to my body has had a positive impact on my mental health—I'm more resilient, and I'm driven to share my learning with others. Thanks for being a part of that by reading this booklet!

BASIC PELVIC NEUROANATOMY

As discussed above, the pelvic girdle anchors the spine. Spinal alignment is important because it supports the spinal cord and all of the important processes the nervous system carries out through the cord. To understand how pain, whether acute or chronic, happens in a particular part of the body, it's important to look back at how the nerves connect that part of the body to the spine.

NEUROMUSCULAR FACTORS AND FUNCTIONING

Nerves branch from the spinal cord to different parts of your pelvis and related structures. Because the layers of your PFM make up a relatively large muscle group, there are multiple nerves that connect to it. The nerves that innervate your pelvic floor stem from your spine starting at your lower lumbars, L4-L5, down through nerves branching from your sacrum, S1-S4. Additionally, the PFM can be affected by nerves coming from your thoracic spine.

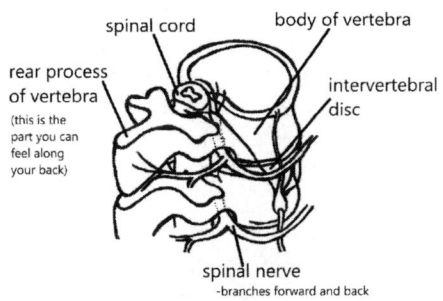

Figure 3.1—Branching of the nerves from a section of the spine. If the spine is not aligned, nerves can easily be pinched. Tight muscles along the spine also affect the nerves and can lead to pain.

Neighboring organs and tissues including the bladder, uterus, vagina, penis, ovaries, testes, and suprarenal gland are all innervated by nerves stemming from the middle of your thoracic spine (where your ribs attach) down to your lumbar vertebrae, T11-L2. The psoas muscle relates to nerves stemming from T12 down to L4, and many functions in the legs, such as the ability to bend the knee or lift the leg, are innervated from the same location as the PFM (Philip, 2016).

Because such a large portion of your spine contributes to the innervation of the PFM and related pelvic anatomy, back pain and pelvic pain can be interrelated. The overlap of nerves means that a problem at one area of the spine can affect an entire region. Because of the way information flows back and forth, the damage and pain to one particular area can end up being felt in another area innervated by the same nerve, a phenomenon known as "referred pain." For example, pelvic pain can become referred pain as it spreads through the abdominal muscles, which are innervated from T7-L2, overlapping with the innervation of the pelvis.

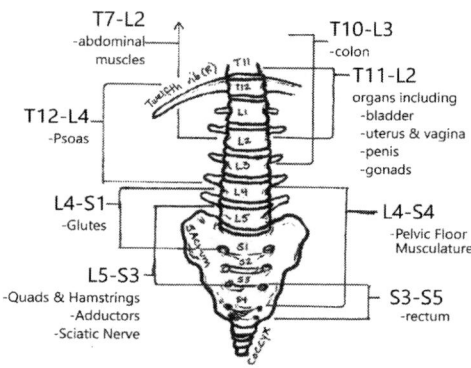

Figure 3.2—A view from the front of the sacrum and lumbar spine. Shows which parts of the spine innervate various muscles, organs, and tissues.

LET'S TALK ABOUT PAIN

Pain is a warning that some structure is damaged or is about to be damaged. When muscles and tissues are stretched, overdistended, or not getting enough oxygen, it triggers nerves called nociceptors, which are specific to sensing pain (Philip, 2016).

The damage that triggers nociceptors may be from one major trauma, such as a vaginal delivery or prostate cancer surgery, or it may have built up over time from ongoing minor traumas such as athletic impacts, heavy lifting, or even just the stretch on joints due to poor postures. In fact, we're seeing an increase in younger people with pelvic pain, which is likely due to higher levels of participation in high impact sports (Bo et al., 2015; Philip, 2016).

When tissue is damaged, it triggers structural and functional changes. Structurally, damage triggers new collagen fibers to form in the tissue. These new fibers are weaker than the original collagen fibers and somewhat "disorganized" (Philip, 2016). It takes time and supportive movement during the healing process for them to organize and strengthen. Scars can also form as part of the healing process. We think of scars as visible marks on our skin, however, soft tissues inside your body can also get scars and adhesions. Just like on your skin, this scar tissue is thick, less elastic, and can even shorten over time (Philip, 2016).

Along with tissue changes, trauma releases neurotransmitters that trigger inflammation and activate certain fibers in the muscles, creating stiffness. Inflammation can also activate a pain response by triggering what are typically called "silent nociceptors" throughout the tissues, joints, and fascia in the area of the damage (Philip, 2016). This activation puts the nerves in a heightened reactive state and can even cause other nerves to spontaneously fire. If the inflammation persists and these nerves are constantly stimulated, it can lead to an increasing amount of pain (Philip, 2016). Hyperalgesia is when the nociceptors are set off by minor/anoxious stimuli. Allodynia is when nociceptors respond to any stimuli at all.

On top of this inflammatory cycle beginning, visceral pain of the internal tissues is uncommon so it can cause confusion in the nervous system. Because our visceral structures don't get pain input on a regular basis, the Central Nervous System (CNS) "mistakes" sensory info from our viscera as superficial damage (Philip, 2016). When I learned this, I understood why my pelvic pain often felt like something external, like a stabbing pain or a bad sunburn on the inside.

Over time, changes that happen to the tissues and nerves as a result of persistent stimulation–such as from inflammation, scarring, or irregular stress like from bad posture or repetitive injuries–can often lead to a level of pain that appears not to match the stimulus. This constant input can change the communication between the nerves and the spine, and cause referred pain. If you've experienced pelvic pain that spreads up through your abs, or back pain that spreads down your leg, you're familiar with referred pain. It's one more thing that makes an accurate diagnosis difficult to make based solely on the location of pain (Philip, 2016).

As a result of expanding and increasing pain, especially when lacking a diagnosis, many sufferers end up avoiding activity, leading to deconditioning of the muscles, reduced function, further damage, and ultimately more pain.

The following is a series of cycles I've adapted from Peter Philip's *Pelvic Pain and Dysfunction* (2016). I found these helpful to understanding how pain builds, what makes it complicated and hard to diagnose, and why gentle movement is key to managing symptoms.

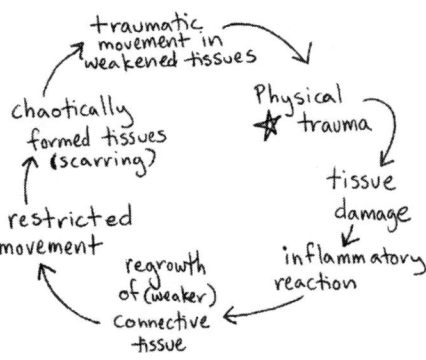

Fig 4.1—How tissue damage can lead to more tissue damage.

As inflammation continues, we add another piece to this cycle. Remember that when pain starts in the inflammation cycle, it often spreads and triggers more pain receptors, leading to referred pain.

People in pain often limit activity in order to minimize the pain. While it's wise to slow down and rest when there's something wrong, complete avoidance of activity leads to weakening in the muscles and surrounding supportive structures. It can also cause a tightening of the fascia, which can be very painful and cause people to take on protective postures, worsening the tightness and weakness. Tight and weakened muscles put more pressure on the joint and other structures resulting in a greater chance of reinjury, more inflammation, and aggravated nerves (Philip, 2016).

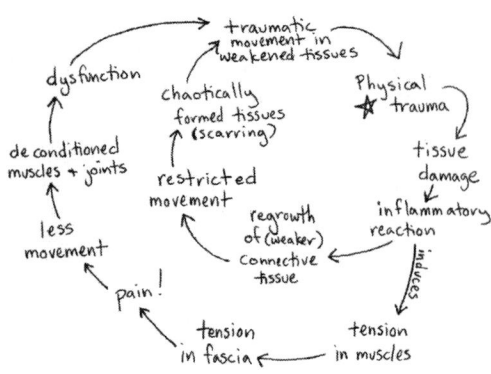

Figure 4.2—The inflammatory reaction initially protects but over time can lead to further dysfunction in damaged tissues. No movement means less nourishment of muscles and connective tissue, which can slow the healing process.

Another common component of pain, especially referred pain, is muscle spasm or hypertonicity. This is when the muscle locks into a tense state. We think this response is an attempt by the body to protect the muscle and joint, however it can be very painful (Philip, 2016). A common example of muscle spasm is a leg cramp or "charley horse," which can be very intense. These often come from overuse, dehydration, or an electrolyte imbalance, but muscle spasms can also be triggered by damage to a joint, often due to a weakened muscle. In addition, while it may feel like a muscle spasm comes on quickly, it's often the result of an overuse injury from repetitive microtraumas, like running and sports on hard surfaces, sustained or repeated movement (including bad posture), or repetitive load (Philip, 2016). These examples are voluntary actions, but the PFM can also experience involuntary repetitive "pelvic bruxing," which is similar to TMJ (temporal-mandibular joint) bruxing, a painful condition in which the jaw muscles are continually clenched.

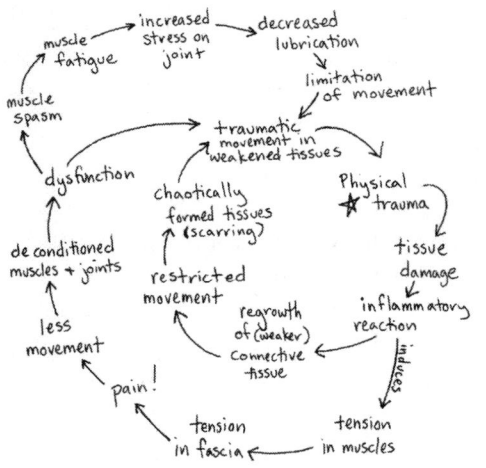

Fig 4.3—Weakened muscles and connective tissue put stress on joints leading to muscle spasm. This condition adds further positive feedback to our cycle with the risk of reinjury and increasing pain.

THE STRESS AND EMOTIONAL PART OF PAIN

Once pain starts, it can become a major player in this cycle from a psychological standpoint. Pain is always subjective (Philip, 2016). As described above, there's a clear physiological reason for this—repeatedly affected nerves amplify pain signals. Anyone who has had chronic pain, or even acute internal pain, can tell you what a drain it is psychologically. The pain might be severe enough to be distracting and the doctor may prescribe pain relievers or muscle relaxers that ease the pain but make it difficult to function, adding to the frustration. Also, visceral internal pain like pelvic pain, "does not accurately reflect the degree of tissue damage" (Philip, 2016). As mentioned above, it's uncommon so it confuses your nociceptors and might feel like something else. This can cause you to perseverate, meaning you just can't stop thinking about the pain. Perhaps you can't stay off the internet trying to diagnose yourself, or you may repeatedly touch the painful area trying to figure it out. While that may help you to be more familiar with that area, it also may further irritate the area.

On top of this, the pain may be causing you stress—whether from the actual pain or from an inability to function as you once did. Stress, both acute and chronic, are known to create an endocrine response, which adds to the inflammatory reaction further contributing to muscle tension, pain, and distress.

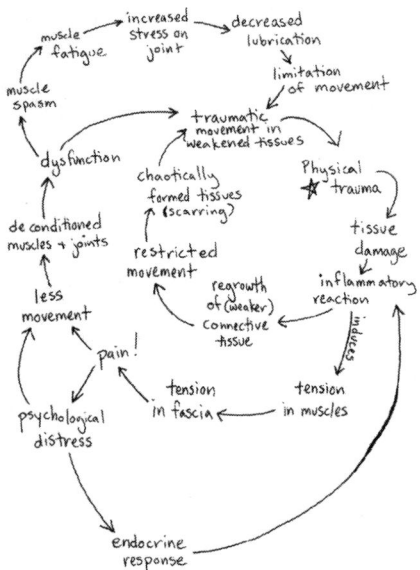

Fig. 4.4—The psychological toll of pain can exacerbate symptoms by contributing to the pain cycle in multiple ways.

As stress (physical and/or emotional) continues, "centralization" can amplify the pain (Philip, 2016). This occurs when conditions such as anxiety, neurosis, or major depression activate the nociceptive pathway of the CNS in a way that mimics the perception of pain. This process is thought to contribute to the increased sympathetic ("fight or flight") activity and decreased parasympathetic ("rest and digest") activity found in sufferers of chronic pain conditions such as fibromyalgia, IBS, migraines, and pelvic pain (Philip, 2016).

The big idea here is that dwelling on the issue and feeling stress related to it can exacerbate pain. This is part of why pain is so complex and often requires the help of multiple practitioners. For those suffering from chronic pain, it can be frustrating to feel like you're bouncing from one professional to another. It helps me to think of these different providers as a team. Modern medicine tends to compartmentalize different issues, so thinking about a team helps pull them together to reach a more holistic understanding of a pain diagnosis. As you see from the above cycles, these factors all feed into each other and cannot be compartmentalized. Along with a medical doctor, it can be helpful to see a physical therapist and a mental health professional, such as someone specializing in cognitive behavioral therapy. Look for providers that work to educate you. Education is empowerment and is key to caring for your body.

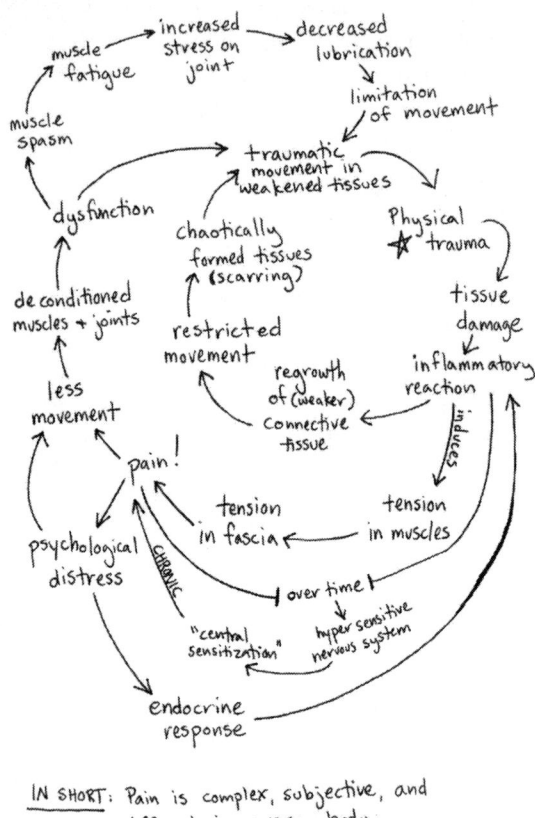

Fig. 4.5—Over time, a constantly stimulated nervous system can become hypersensitive, leading to chronic pain. Pain is complex, subjective, and different in every body.

MOVEMENTS TO SUPPORT AND CARE FOR YOUR PELVIC FLOOR

IMPORTANT NOTE: If you are having any pain, discomfort, or other issues, it's essential to get guidance from a healthcare practitioner, and I don't just mean a physical therapist on YouTube. There are some great PT videos, but they can't tell you if you're doing something wrong, or even moving in a way that will make your situation worse. A physical therapist will start by assessing the main issue. Whether it's injury, tension, or atrophy will require different approaches. To help you make real progress, and do so without causing further injury, a PT can create a tailored program and provide the biofeedback essential for success.

MOVEMENT IN A HEALTHY PELVIC FLOOR

A healthy pelvic floor is like a trampoline. It supports your organs and when pushed on by the abs or pulled on by other muscles, it responds by contracting to give a little pushback. If the PFM has sustained damage, whether in one traumatic event or due to minor stresses over time, it's "like a trampoline that's lost its bounce"—it can't push back, and so when pushed on, just gets stretched further (Bo et al., 2015).

Remember, the PFM is largely made up of skeletal muscle attached to your pelvic girdle, so can be addressed like any other muscle. Gentle and supportive movements are clinically proven to maintain a healthy body and to support healing in damaged tissues. Movement stimulates nourishment of the muscles and joints. In healing tissues, gentle movement can reduce tight restrictions and scarring and support communication between muscles and nerves, improving function and preventing a hypersensitive or dysfunctional pain response (Philip, 2016).

RELEASING HELD TENSION

Before we begin to talk about movement and strengthening, it's important to address that many pelvic issues (and pain in general) come from built up tension over time. The stresses of daily life cause us to hold extra tension in our bodies. Many of us also spend long hours sitting and we may either neglect to move our bodies or we engage in intense exercise as an attempt to counteract that sitting. Some of us have particular traumas—physical, emotional, or both—that we are holding in our PFM. Perhaps damage or weakness has caused other muscles to overcompensate. Trying to strengthen damaged muscles or force "proper" posture on already taxed muscles that aren't in alignment can exacerbate problems and trigger painful spasms and other neuromuscular issues. Getting in touch with our bodies to find where we're holding this tension allows us to intentionally release the muscles, which can improve strength training and prevent further damage.

My PT noted that my Psoas was especially tight. In search of other approaches, I came across a video by Martha Peterson (Essential Somatics, 2019). It was a simple exercise and my introduction to Clinical Somatic Education, a movement practice with roots in Somatics, Feldenkrais, and Alexander Technique, among others. All of these movement practices center on taking time to become more aware of your body. You begin by noticing tension and then use gentle movements to "remind" the body of its natural alignment and function, including how the muscles should relax. The simple approach was revolutionary for me. I began a nightly practice that begins with lying on my back on the floor doing a "Soma Scan," which is just taking 2-3 minutes to be still and notice where your body is holding tension. This simple practice is a great way to get in touch with your body and get feedback. You might notice as you move throughout the day how you hold yourself or move in ways that contribute to where you feel tightness and pain.

Breath practice is another way to get in touch with your body and give feedback to the relaxation system. Many of us only take shallow breaths into our chests. One of the reasons for this is that we're holding tension in our abs and back. You can train yourself to breathe more deeply by taking time to intentionally take deeper breaths that fill the space down into your belly. Breath practice is the main component to this short series of pelvic opening exercises adapted from *Women's Running* (Levy, 2020).

1. **Abdominal breathing/3-part breathing**—Lie on your back with your knees bent, placing one hand on your chest and one on your abdomen. Breathe in slowly to fill your lungs and allow your diaphragm to fill your belly. Keep opening, moving the breath down into your pelvic floor. Slowly release your breath from each of these three areas. Repeat for 2-5 minutes.

2. **Breathing into Child's Pose**—Kneel down and fold forward with your forehead resting on the ground. If that's not comfortable, stack your

hands and rest your forehead on them, or use a small pillow. Inhale slowly and imagine the back of your shirt expanding as you breathe into your ribs, opening down into your PFM.

3. **Abdominal lengthening**—Lie face down with legs extended and hands by your shoulders. Press away from the floor to gently lift your torso up until your arms are straight. Your hips should remain on the ground. Relax your abs and back as you take three deep breaths in this position. Lower again and repeat 2-5 times. If you feel *any* strain in your back or abs, you can do this propped on your elbows rather than with arms fully extended.

4. **Hip opening**—Lie on your back with your knees bent and place one foot on the opposite knee. Lift the bottom leg and take hold of it around the thigh with your hands. Take three deep abdominal breaths in this position. Repeat with the other leg. When you do this, remember to think of "opening" and "length" rather than trying to "stretch" anything.

LENGTHEN, DON'T STRETCH (A PERSONAL STORY OF PT AND PAIN)

A lot of experts, including my physical therapist, discuss stretching as a way to release tight muscles. While *gentle* stretching can warm up muscles before a workout, giving a strong stretch to tight or otherwise damaged muscles can actually be problematic. Remember earlier when I talked about what happens during trauma? That can happen from stretching too. Overstretching, even when it's causing that "good pain," can act as a form of trauma on the tissue, which kicks in your body's inflammatory response (Philip, 2016). When tissue is damaged, the fascia and other connective tissue that replaces the damaged tissue is stiffer and needs to become organized. Too much mechanical force from intense stretching or even treatments that attempt to treat the connective tissue fascia by stretching may actually cause more fascial tightness and pain. The stiff, sensitive tissue is being reinjured, triggering the muscle cells in a way that furthers inflammation and pain (Philip, 2016).

I learned this truth about overstretching the hard way, after experiencing serious crying-on-the-couch level pain for several days after some of my physical therapy sessions. Stretching exercises had been given to me, and I dutifully followed them. At the time, I didn't know about this stretch response—I thought I had just overdone it and was surprised at how little it took to overdo it. On top of that, the therapist was using heat and ultrasound therapy (deep heat) to stimulate my muscles and get them to relax. I later learned this was the opposite of what I needed.

To explain, if you look back at the cycles from earlier (pg. 24), you'll see that my muscles were tight due to damage—they were weak and in the healing process—they had contracted into a spasm in some unconscious protective act of my nervous system. When I stretched, trying to loosen them, my body just interpreted it as more trauma, going into further protective mode. Then when we added heat, we were really just adding inflammation. My body was thrown into a positive feedback loop which I felt as more and more intense pain. Lessons learned—ice is my best friend when in pain, and while I still do my "stretching exercises," I focus on lengthening and alignment and I

> never stretch with any kind of force. Gentle movement is key to caring for your body.

READY TO MOVE? START WITH ISOLATION

Many of us have heard of a Kegel. In contemporary culture, they're recommended like some kind of vaginal panacea. In fact, after I had my son, I told my midwife that things didn't feel right, that it seemed like the front wall of my vagina was falling in. While what I was describing was a bladder prolapse, I was told things would soon "snap back" into place, ". . . just do some Kegels." I did some Kegels, but since I hadn't been offered any instruction by my midwife (or anyone prior), I stopped doing them. I never felt like I was doing them right, not to mention I was struggling to feel a contraction because I likely had muscle and nerve damage to my levator ani after birthing a child with a huge head. I've now learned that it was probably for the better that I stopped, because doing Kegels the wrong way can actually make issues worse, particularly if you have a prolapse (Philip, 2016).

The very first step before you can strengthen or support your PFM is to ensure you can do an isolated PFM contraction. In 1952, Dr. Kegel published an article in which he described a PFM contraction having two components: a squeeze around pelvic openings and an inward lift (Bo et al., 2015). When we are told to "do kegels" we often don't even have this much information. A study by Bump in 1991 showed that brief verbal instruction was not enough in teaching proper PFM contraction technique for 50% of the women they studied. In fact, 25% of the study participants contracted in a way that created a downward pressure on the bladder rather than the desired lifting effect (Kisner, 2018).

There are several factors that make a voluntary PFM contraction difficult to perform. Kari Bo et al. (2015) explain that the PFM has an "invisible" location inside the pelvis; "neither men nor women have ever learned to contract the PFM and most people would be unaware of the automatic contractions of the muscles." The muscles are also small, which from a neurophysiological perspective, makes them more difficult to contract. A lot of people also push while they are on the toilet. This involves your PFM muscles, but it is the opposite action of what you're trying to get them to do in order to strengthen them, making it even more difficult for people who have that habit. If the PFM is weak, especially if there's been damage, there may be less sensation and only the ability to perform low intensity contractions, which don't provide much biofeedback. Without biofeedback the body is not triggering the reflex to contract against pressure, which is what prevents leakage of urine (Bo et al., 2015). While I've mostly focused on support and managing pelvic pain, incontinence is actually one of the main reasons people see a physical therapist who specializes in the pelvic floor. I'll discuss this more in the section on Activities of Daily Life.

But in the first section you made the point that the PFM doesn't operate in isolation. Why do you want me to isolate it?

If you start training without first learning to do an isolated PFM contraction, there can be too much recruitment of the larger and more commonly used muscle groups, which can mask the awareness and strength of the PFM contraction (Bo et al., 2015). You may feel like you're performing a strong contraction, but it may be the abs or glutes that are actually creating it, not the PFM.

Recruiting the other muscles without first strengthening the PFM can put added pressure on the PFM, which may stretch and weaken the muscles, as well as damaging the connective tissues and increasing the risk of developing pelvic organ prolapse (Bo et al., 2015).

By isolating your PFM, you're also further educating yourself about what it does. Because we often don't think about it until a problem develops, intentionally familiarizing yourself with them is essential to being able to support, strengthen, and heal the PFM. Clinicians have found that muscle training in how to do an isolated PFM contraction is valuable regardless of the patient's issue or cause of symptoms (Kisner, 2018). If nothing else, it helps people become more familiar with their PFM and its role in daily activities.

OK, I get it, so how do I do an isolated PFM Contraction?

The simplest way to think about contracting your PFM in isolation is to think about lift. You'll sometimes hear references to doing a kegel as "just contract like you're trying to stop your urine." While that contraction is done by the PFM, trying to stop your urine is not natural and is not helpful because you could end up putting pressure downward, which causes problems as outlined above.

Start by lying on your back. This removes the pressure of gravity while you learn to isolate your PFM. Visualize that "basket" of muscles and interwoven ligaments and fascia that make up the PFM (Mulligan, 2013). Imagine you're lifting up the base of the basket as you contract your PFM.

Because your PFM has 3 layers, you can also think about what each of them does by contracting in a 3-step process. Think "pinch," "squeeze," "elevate." Saying these words out loud can help make sure you're breathing normally as you contract (Kisner, 2018). Don't breathe out hard while doing a contraction, because that puts added downward pressure, and you want to be lifting. If you can't feel the difference between the "pinch," "squeeze," and "elevate," try propping up your hips on a couple of pillows to further take pressure off of your PFM. Once your PFM gets stronger you can remove the pillows, and eventually you'll continue strengthening by doing this standing.

IDEAS TO VISUALIZE WHAT YOUR PFM IS DOING DURING ISOLATION:

- It is a hammock and you're pulling up to flatten the bottom of it (Mulligan, 2013).
- It is a basket and becomes more tightly woven as you contract (Mulligan, 2013).
- You have a string coming out of your belly button. When you slowly pull it, it lifts your pelvic floor (Mulligan, 2013).
- You're holding or sitting on a marble and pulling it in (Kisner, 2018).
- Your PFM is an elevator lifting from floor to floor (Kisner, 2018).

Once you feel like you have the hang of it, you can do a short set of PFM contractions. A sequence recommended by Carolyn Kisner et al. in *Therapeutic Exercise: Foundations and Techniques* (2018) has three stages:

1. Start with a few rounds of contracting and relaxing. Hold each contraction for 3-5 seconds. Repeat 10 times. Counting out loud while you do this can help to keep breathing normal. Make sure you're not recruiting other muscles, and don't use a strong breath out with contraction (that only adds pressure).

2. Follow this with a few quick contractions, about 15-20, while breathing normally. The quick contractions help with type II fiber response, which withstands pressure (like from coughing).

3. Then you can do an "elevator" lift. Imagine an elevator going up and down from floor to floor as you contract in a smooth gradual lifting and lowering of the PFM. Make sure you fully relax between contractions by imagining the elevator going all the way to the basement. Keep your breathing slow and deep as you complete this exercise.

If there is any weakness or tension, the above routine may be overdoing it. And overdoing it can lead to spasms and other complications. If it feels like too much, see a medical professional to make sure there aren't other issues. It's fine to start with a shortened version of this. Starting with light contractions and increasing the time between contractions can help strengthen without increasing tension (Kisner, 2018).

If a person is experiencing prolapse or atrophy, doing this with hips propped up or on all fours can help take pressure off of the pelvic floor while working to strengthen it (Kisner, 2018). Focusing on a rhythmic contraction of each layer ("pinch," "squeeze," "elevate") can also make sure you're strengthening in a way that is supportive and not adding pressure (Kisner, 2018).

I COULD DO THIS ALL DAY! WAIT, SHOULD I DO THIS ALL DAY?

One other piece that complicates PFM education is conflicting advice on how much conditioning to do per day. In 1956, Dr. Kegel recommended performing at least 500 contractions per day (Bo et al., 2015)! I had a gynecologist recently tell me the gold standard was 10 contractions 10x per day. These both seem like a lot, and based on more modern strength training studies, more repetitions do not improve strength. Bo et al. state that, "Performing many repetitions with very light resistance will result in no or minimal strength gain . . . Fewer contractions take less time and may therefore also be much more motivating. Hence exercise adherence may increase" (Bo et al., 2015).

My PT also supported the idea that doing less with better form was ideal—the most important thing is that you're doing them right and doing them at least once a day. Ultimately, whatever the amount *you actually do* is the amount that is best.

MOTOR RELEARNING DEPENDS ON SENSORY FEEDBACK OR *"AM I DOING THIS RIGHT?"*

Even with these tips, it can take some time and practice to be able to perform controlled and coordinated PFM contractions. Many of us are not aware of our PFM in the first place, nor have we tried to contract it voluntarily, so we are unable to hold the contraction or perform repetitive or strong contractions during our first attempts. It can also take time because part of training your muscles is teaching the nervous system (Bo et al., 2015).

The good news is, there are some easy ways to get biofeedback to teach your nervous system and give you the confidence to keep up a routine. Another term for the feedback you're getting is neuromuscular re-education. This component is essential because there are often sensory deficits, and when working on conditioning or re-conditioning muscles, motor learning happens. The feedback provides sensation that promotes retention of those motor learning pathways (Kisner, 2018).

Start by getting familiar with the pelvis. You learned about the anatomy in part one of this booklet, and you felt how it relates to alignment in part two (see "Try This" on pg 14). Start each session of training by moving your pelvis slowly in different directions. You'll gain a better understanding of the PFM as you pay attention to how the movement feels, as well as how the alignment shifts, what other muscles become engaged, and where you might be holding tension in those muscles (Bo et al., 2015).

Moving on to the PFM contractions, the most effective and accurate biofeedback is from a good physical therapist who can feel your muscles, provide you with touch feedback, both internally and externally, and direct you through exercises while giving you a good sense of what's happening in your PFM and what you should be focusing on (certain areas that are tight, overall weakness, etc). In my experience, I had a huge jump in strength after just one week of doing proper PFM contractions guided by the PT. It was too quick for this to be just about strength, but showed that my body was starting to learn how to get those muscles to work together.

You can still get some good biofeedback on your own by placing your fingers on your perineum as you do a PFM contraction. You should feel that you are lifting up and away from your fingers, rather than any pushing down. If you're comfortable with it, you can even use a mirror to see the lifting movement of the perineum and/or scrotum (Bo et al., 2015). Also try putting a hand on your lower abdomen as you contract your PFM. This will make sure that you're not recruiting your abdominal muscles while working to isolate your PFM.

Another simple biofeedback exercise you can do is to sit on an armrest or at the edge of a table with your legs spread apart slightly, feet on the floor, and back straight. You should be able to feel the armrest against your perineum, which will provide feedback. Then perform a PFM contraction by squeezing and lifting your perineum away from the armrest or table without rising up or pressing down on your feet (Bo et al., 2015).

Along with gentle touch by yourself or from a professional, there are other tools you can use. Pelvic weights, such as stone eggs have become popular. These can be helpful for biofeedback, but it is not recommended to keep them in for extended periods of time. Walking around with them, as is sometimes advised, means keeping your PFM in contraction. This can rob it of oxygen and lead to reduced blood flow and painful spasms (Bo et al., 2015). There are also pelvic floor trainers. Some even hook up to apps on your phone where you squeeze to play games. My concern is they may be distracting you from being fully aware of what's going on, however seeing, for example, a butterfly go higher as you squeeze harder is strong biofeedback, particularly for visual learners. Some of these trainers also have sensors at shallow and deep levels to give you an idea of how fully you're contracting your PFM, and to make sure you're focusing on different layers.

Here is a list of common mistakes to watch out for when learning to perform a PFM contraction (Bo et al., 2015):

- Contraction of outer abdominal muscles instead of the PFM—Notice whether your back is curving or there is any tucking the stomach inwards.

- Contraction of hip adductor muscles instead of the PFM—Your inner thighs should stay relaxed as you learn to isolate your PFM.

- Contraction of the gluteal muscles instead of the PFM—You may notice your butt lift up from the floor if you're pressing your glutes together.

- Holding your breath—Keep breathing as regularly as possible. Counting out loud or saying "pinch, squeeze, elevate" as you contract can help keep your breathing regular.

- Enhanced inhaling—Some people inhale deeply and engage their abs thinking they're lifting up the PFM.

- Straining or pressing downwards—This sometimes happens during strong exhalation and will put pressure on the PFM. Think lift!

PFM SUPPORT DURING ACTIVITIES OF DAILY LIFE

Once you feel like you are performing a PFM contraction correctly it's important to also start including PFM isolations in your Activities of Daily Life (ADLs). Using effective PFM contractions before activities like lifting, standing up, or coughing, can help support and protect the PFM, while also providing some of the biofeedback/NM re-education your body needs to help encourage the regular and automatic engagement of the PFM during these and other activities. As part of re-education, engaging your PFM during ADLs will also help encourage coordination of the PFM with related muscles; stabilizing the trunk, engaging the transverse abdominal muscle, the diaphragm, and the multifidus muscles of your lower back (Junginger, 2014).

If there is any damage to the PFM it can keep the muscles from functioning properly and working together. With damage and subsequent atrophy, there also may be less sensation in the PFM muscles, meaning that getting biofeedback is essential. Working to intentionally engage your PFM through ADLs and regular movement helps re-train the neuromuscular reactions and sensations.

Whether or not there's been damage, changes in the body over time mean incontinence is a common issue in men and women. A 2014 study found that incorporating PFM contractions into ADLs can prevent urinary leakage (Junginger, 2014). They instructed patients in PFM contraction and termed this movement "The Knack." They asked participants to maintain a submaximal PFM contraction during breathing, urgency, and on the way to the toilet, and to pre-contract before coughing, lifting, blowing the nose, etc. They found that this practice didn't just help strengthen, but "taught correct and selective muscle contractions that elevate the bladder and support coordination of muscle functions" (Junginger, 2014). Similar to my earlier strength training example, the study found that the patients had success within one week, which is too soon to be due to muscle strength itself, and could show that getting instruction and biofeedback on how to properly engage your PFM makes a big difference in being able to do so (Junginger, 2014).

MOVING ON AND INCORPORATING MORE MUSCLES

Once you've gotten the hang of a proper PFM isolation, you can move onto other conditioning. The big goal is to recondition without any straining (Philip, 2016). This will take time. Go slow. And again, if anything hurts or doesn't feel right, seek out a professional who can evaluate your condition and give you specific tools to address it.

Because the PFM is made up of skeletal muscles it will adapt to strength training the same way as other skeletal muscles. Strength training can increase muscle mass, tone, and response. However, in order to continue strength training you'll need to continue to increase load and engagement (Bo et al., 2015). You can start this simply by working up to stronger, more fully engaged PFM contractions.

Another way to increase load is by doing contractions in different positions, such as standing upright, which adds the force of gravity. Performing PFM contractions while lunging or squatting adds load from different angles, coordinating with a variety of muscles. According to Philip, the most challenging position is holding a PFM contraction while performing a free-standing squat (Philip, 2016).

If you're into gadgets, you can also increase load through the use of weights or pelvic floor exercisers, as mentioned in the section on biofeedback. Again, there are some differences of opinion on whether or not these are effective and/or safe to use. Along with the concerns about misuse, such as the practice of holding them in for extended periods of time (hello, cramps) or even sleeping with them in (hello, bacterial infection), practitioners have concerns that some of them may be difficult to use, making them ineffective or causing people to give up using them (Bo et al., 2015). If you want to try one of these products, look for ones made of medical-grade silicone, as porous stone can attract bacteria, and don't use it beyond a typical PFM routine, like the simple 3-part routine discussed earlier. If you're interested in trying these or you have any questions about them, talk to your medical professional.

Along with training and strengthening the PFM itself, you'll need to retrain the muscle groups that support it. The abdominal muscles, hip muscles, low back muscles, and inner thighs all play a role in PFM functioning and there can be muscular imbalance, postural issues, and generalized weakness contributing to pelvic and back issues. To protect itself, the PFM should co-contract when any of these muscle groups are engaged. If there is dysfunction in the PFM and no co-contraction when you engage your abs, for example, it puts downward pressure, overloading and stretching the PFM (Bo et al., 2015). Relearning to coordinate PFM contractions with other muscles will help protect your PFM, and, even more importantly, it will reinforce neuromuscular learning as you strengthen the "basket" in all directions (Kisner, 2018).

Once you can regularly perform a proper isolation of the PFM, you can add additional actions such as holding the contraction through a few deep diaphragmatic breaths, and then holding the contraction as you lift your hips up into a bridge or do an abdominal crunch. Make sure to relax fully after each set of these actions (Philip, 2016). Going slowly and intentionally engaging the PFM as you start adding additional muscle groups will help re-educate your PFM to automatically contract when you engage other muscle groups. This is essential to supporting and protecting your PFM as you further condition neighboring muscle groups.

As you develop a PFM routine, no exercises should hurt beyond typical muscle fatigue. Like we saw in the earlier cycles, pain begets pain (Philip, 2016). If you find yourself developing pain within 48 hours after doing exercise, you are either doing too much and could be triggering muscle spasms or you need to see a medical professional to address an underlying issue. This is your body saying slow down. However, don't stop. Movement is so important to reconditioning. You may have to go very slowly and return to gentle releasing exercises or adding props such as a pillow under the hips. Keep in mind that no matter where you are in your journey, or what your fitness level, doing gentle movements helps care for your body and support neuromuscular functioning and coordination.

IN SUMMARY

*E*ducation is empowerment! Learning about your body and paying attention to it are key to taking care of it.

Your pelvic floor is a complex and layered set of muscles, ligaments, and fascia that spans the pelvic girdle. Because of its location at the base of your spine, and its coordination with other muscles, it's particularly prone to developing pain and dysfunction. Education about the pelvic floor and posture has been clinically proven to help those suffering from pain (Philip, 2016). Managing symptoms can be complex and require an integrated approach involving assessment, education, biofeedback, and addressing mental health.

To strengthen and support your pelvic floor, you'll need to know that a PFM contraction (fka Kegel) involves two parts: lift and squeeze. Approach conditioning slowly and make sure you're getting biofeedback to help the muscles and nerves learn to coordinate. A good physical therapist is a great resource for this. To support and care for your pelvic floor and your body as a whole, keep learning and move gently every day.

REFERENCES

Bo, Kari, et al. *Evidence-based Physical Therapy for the Pelvic Floor: Bridging science and clinical practice.* Elsevier, 2015.

[Essential Somatics]. (2019, February 1). *The Best Psoas Release* [video file]. Retrieved from youtube.com/watch?v=91ViRjiDOO8

Junginger, Baerbel, Elisa Seibt, and Kaven Baessler. *Bladder-neck effective, integrative pelvic floor rehabilitation program: follow-up investigation.* European Journal of Obstetrics & Gynecology and Reproductive Biology, 174 (2014), pp. 150-153.

Levy, Kathryn. (2020, April 13). *Do These 4 Moves to Relax Tight Pelvic Floor Muscles.*

Retrieved from womensrunning.com/health/4-moves-loosen-tight-pelvic-floor/

Kisner, Carolyn, et al. *Therapeutic Exercise: Foundations and Technique.* 7th ed., F. A. Davis, 2018.

Mulligan, Tasha. (2013) *Posture Must Be Consistent.* Retrieved from hab-it.com/posture-must-be-consistent

Open Hand Health. (2021, January 23). F A S C I A [Instagram post]. Retrieved from instagram.com/p/CKZrZkrhkdK/?igshid=8z551gzsjpnd

Philip, Peter A. *Pelvic Pain and Dysfunction: A Differential Diagnosis Manual.* Thieme, 2016.

RESOURCES I LIKE

PELVIC HEALTH
- Brianne Grogan, DPT, femfusionfitness.com/
- Pelvic Health Rehabilitation Center: Information is spread throughout site, and the blog has a lot of good resources, pelvicpainrehab.com/blog/
- Sara Reardon, DPT, @TheVaginaWhisperer, thevagwhisperer.com
- Tasha Mulligan, PT, hab-it.com

BODY LITERACY AND SEXUAL HEALTH
- All Bodies Health, https://allbodies.com/
- Open Hand Health, IG @openhandhealth
- The Sex Ed, @TheSexEd, TheSexEd.com

EMBODIED MOVEMENT
- Martha Peterson, essentialsomatics.com
- Miranda Esmonde-White: Classical stretch and full body fitness for every age, essentrics.com
- Laura Beth Wenger, @laura.beth.wenger, laurabethwenger.com
- Bernadette Pleasant, theemotionalinstitute.com
- Sequencewiz.org. This site is yoga centric, but it has some excellent imagery and resources on how different postures and poses impact your anatomy and functioning.
- The Shift Network, theshiftnetwork.com, Some of their programs are a little out there, but annually they host free virtual summits in Somatic Movement, Breathwork, and more.

There are more and more resources out there. I'm sure there are others that can help that I haven't even come across. If you have a resource you like and want to recommend please comment and share through social media @GoSlowStudio or send me a message at GoSlowStudio@gmail.com

GLOSSARY

ADLs (Activities of Daily Life): As it sounds, this refers to activities an individual does throughout the day. Your PFM naturally engages during all kinds of activities you do.

atrophy: A gradual decline in functionality due to underuse or neglect; in body tissues and organs, reflects loss of mass and strength.

biofeedback: The process of gaining greater awareness of physiological functions of one's own body; may be used as a way to learn to self-regulate or to re-establish neuromuscular functioning in damaged tissues.

collagen: The main structural protein in the extracellular matrix found in the body's connective tissues; It is the most abundant protein in mammals and is found in cartilage, bones, tendons, ligaments, skin, blood vessels, etc.

CNS (Central Nervous System): The part of the nervous system consisting primarily of the brain and spinal cord.

deconditioned: A reduction in muscle mass and strength as the result of decreased physical activity.

fascia: Thin bands or sheets of connective tissue, primarily made of collagen, that attach, stabilize, enclose, and separate muscles and other internal organs; largely made of collagen fibers arranged in a way that makes them flexible in certain directions.

incontinence: The involuntary loss of urine or fecal matter.

innervated/innervation: The way in which nerves stem from the spinal cord to the tissues; can also refer to how a signal from the nervous system is supplied to the tissues.

ischemic: Lacking the oxygen that is needed to keep cells alive; may also lead to reduction in cells' ability to receive nutrients and get rid of wastes.

nociceptors: Pain receptors; nerves that respond to damaging or potentially damaging stimuli by sending signals to the spinal cord and brain, which are interpreted as pain.

neuromuscular re-education: Consists of training (or re-training) your muscles, your brain, and the nerves used for them to communicate with each other to improve movement, strength, balance, and function.

NM (neuromuscular): Relating to nerves and muscles and the connection between them.

parasympathetic: Relating to the part of the autonomic nervous system that's responsible for stimulation of the "rest-and-digest" response, which includes activities that occur when the body is at rest, such as digestion, regulating heart rate, and sexual arousal. Its actions are complementary to the sympathetic nervous system, which is responsible for the "fight-or-flight" response.

perineum: Can generally refer to the region between pubic bone and tailbone, and can specifically refer to the surface between the scrotum/vagina and anus.

PFM (Pelvic Floor Musculature): Several layers of muscles that sit within the pelvic girdle of the skeleton, spanning from the pubic bone in front, back to the tailbone, and bordered by the sitting bones. The pelvic floor muscles support the pelvic organs, resist abdominal pressure, and work as sphincters, opening and closing the urethra, rectum, and vagina.

physiological: Relating to the way in which a living organism or bodily part functions.

prolapse: A displacement of a part or organ of the body from its normal position, usually downward or outward; e.g. In a uterine prolapse, the uterus has lost the support of the PFM and connective tissues and slips down into the vaginal cavity, sometimes to the point that it protrudes from the vagina.

referred pain: Pain perceived at a location other than the site of the painful stimulus.

sacrum: A triangular bone in the lower back formed from fused vertebrae and situated between the two hip bones of the pelvis (see figures 2.1 and 2.2).

superficial and deep: These two anatomical terms relate to one another; superficial means more toward the surface of the body and deep means more toward the core of the body.

sympathetic: See parasympathetic.

trauma: A distressing or disturbing experience; may be an emotional shock following a stressful event or physical injury, or, as in medicine, it can refer to the physical injury itself.

viscera: The internal organs in the main cavities of the body, especially those in the abdomen, such as the intestines.

voluntary and involuntary: In the body, voluntary refers to action that is normally controlled by an individual's will, and involuntary refers to automatic responses not controlled by the individual, such as the control of heart rate, blood vessels, and digestion.

ABOUT THE AUTHOR

Amy Wanner Jeansonne works in an academic library and is a former Biology and Environmental Science teacher. This booklet is her first publication as an informal educator. Amy is currently developing Go Slow Studio as a place to explore and share her interests in somatic movement and body-mind education. She lives in Troy, NY with her partner and son.

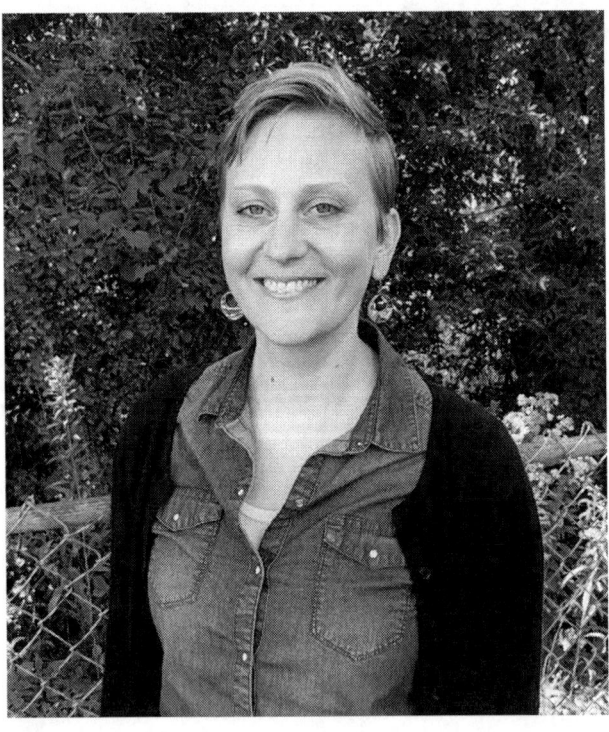